Let's Get Healthy

ur
eth

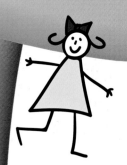

Let's Get Healthy

Your Teeth

Sarah Ridley

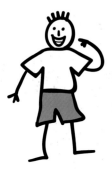

W
FRANKLIN WATTS
LONDON • SYDNEY

This edition first published in 2008 by Franklin Watts.

Franklin Watts
338 Euston Road
London
NW1 3BH

Franklin Watts Australia
Level 17/207 Kent Street
Sydney NSW 2000

Let's Get Healthy is a reduced text version of *Look After Yourself!*
The original texts were by Claire Llewellyn.

Dewey number: 613.2
ISBN: 978 0 7496 8321 4

Printed in China

Franklin Watts is a division of Hachette Children's Books,
an Hachette Livre UK company.
www.hachettelivre.co.uk

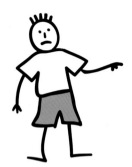

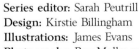

Series editor: Sarah Peutrill
Design: Kirstie Billingham
Illustrations: James Evans
Photographs: Ray Moller unless otherwise acknowledged
Picture research: Diana Morris
Series consultant: Lynn Huggins-Cooper
Dental consultant: Darren Cromey, BDS

Acknowledgments:
Paul Barton/Corbisstockmarket: 25tr.
Rick Gomez/Corbisstockmarket: 15t.
Dr. Peter Gordon/Science Photo Library: 24.
Dr. H.C. Robinson/Science Photo Library: 25b.

With thanks to our models: Aaron, Charlotte, Connor,
Jake and Nadine.

Contents

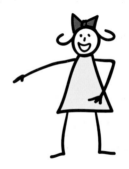

Looking at teeth

Everyone has teeth.

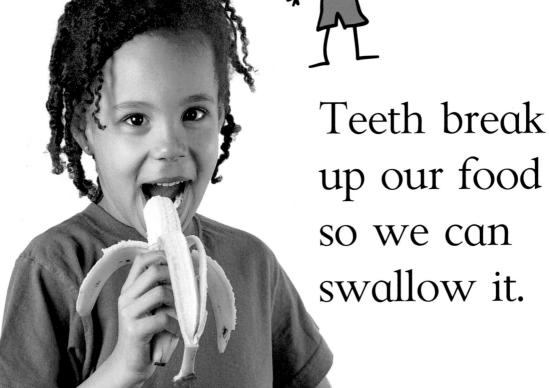

Look in your mouth!

Teeth break up our food so we can swallow it.

Teeth also help us talk – and smile.

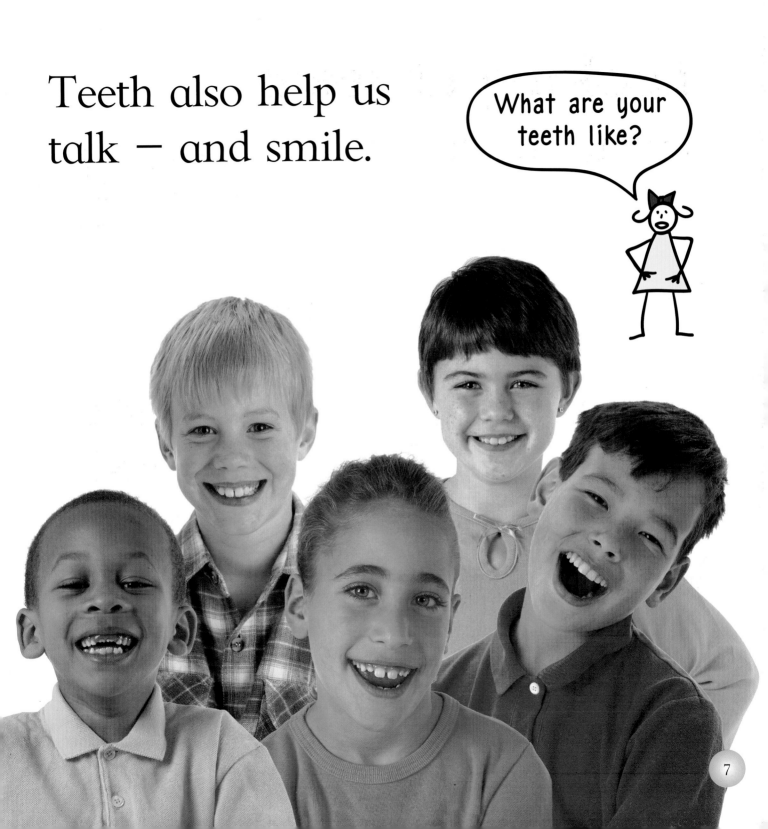

What are your teeth like?

Teeth and gums

Teeth have a strong, white coating called enamel.

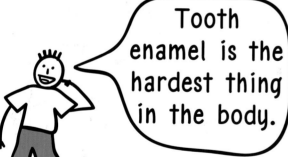

Tooth enamel is the hardest thing in the body.

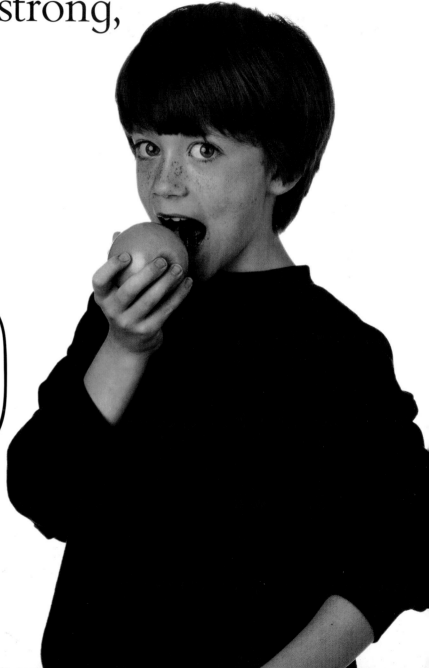

The soft, pink gums help to hold the teeth in place.

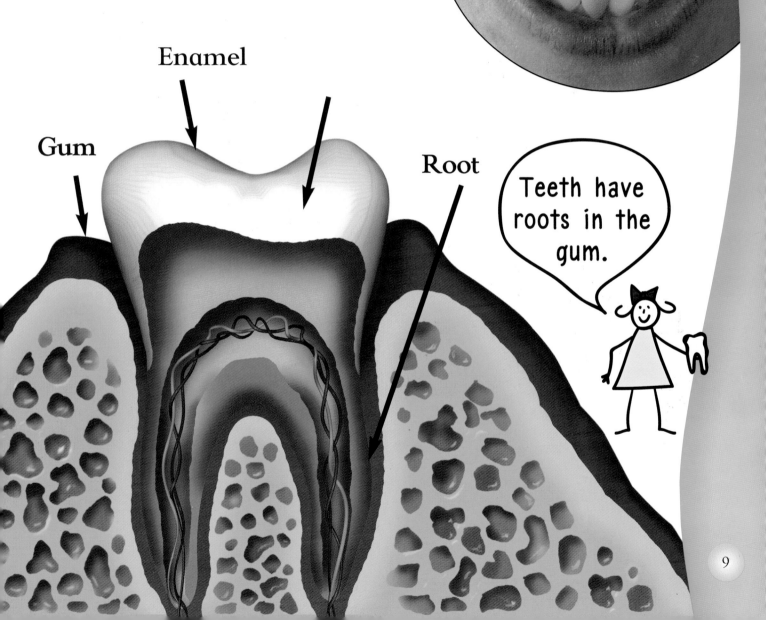

Gum

Enamel

Root

Teeth have roots in the gum.

All sorts of teeth

We have different kinds of teeth.

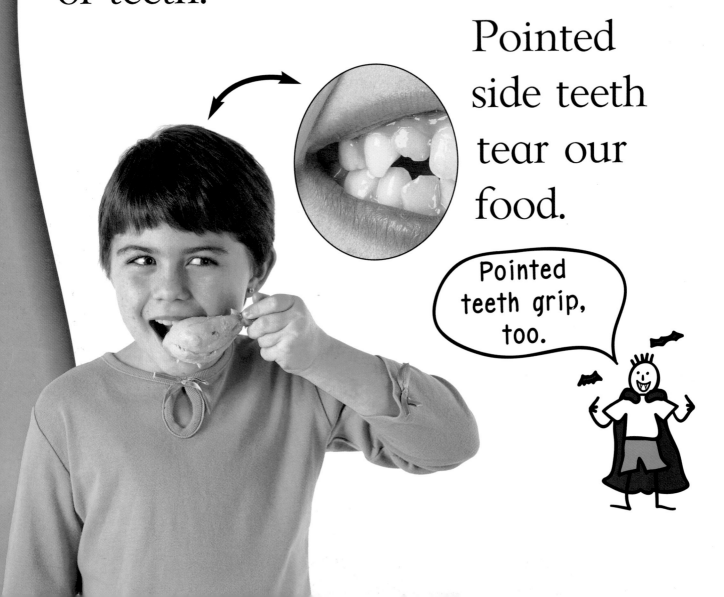

Pointed side teeth tear our food.

Pointed teeth grip, too.

Straight
front teeth
are good
for cutting.

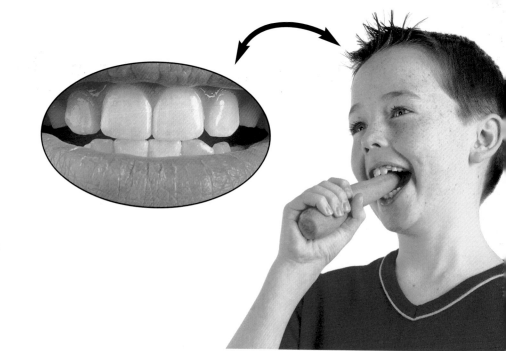

Back teeth
chew.

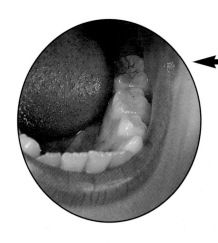

Our teeth
let us eat
all sorts of
food.

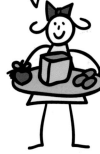

Milk teeth

Milk, or baby, teeth start to grow out of our gums when we are six months old.

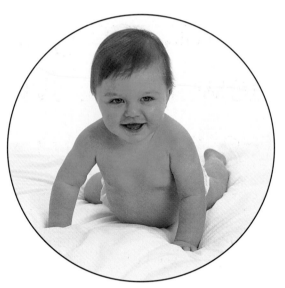

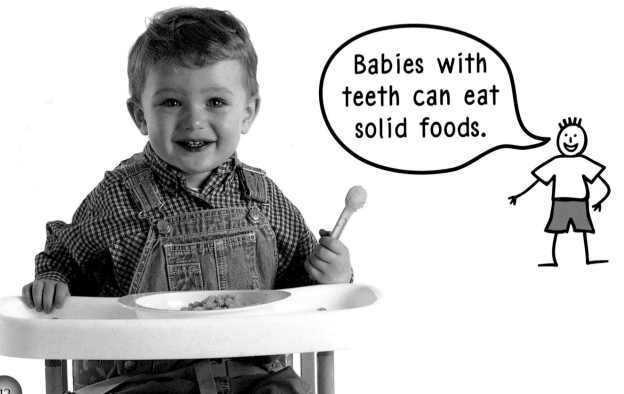

Babies with teeth can eat solid foods.

At about the age of six, we grow new teeth. Milk teeth start to drop out. Adult teeth take their place.

Have you lost a tooth?

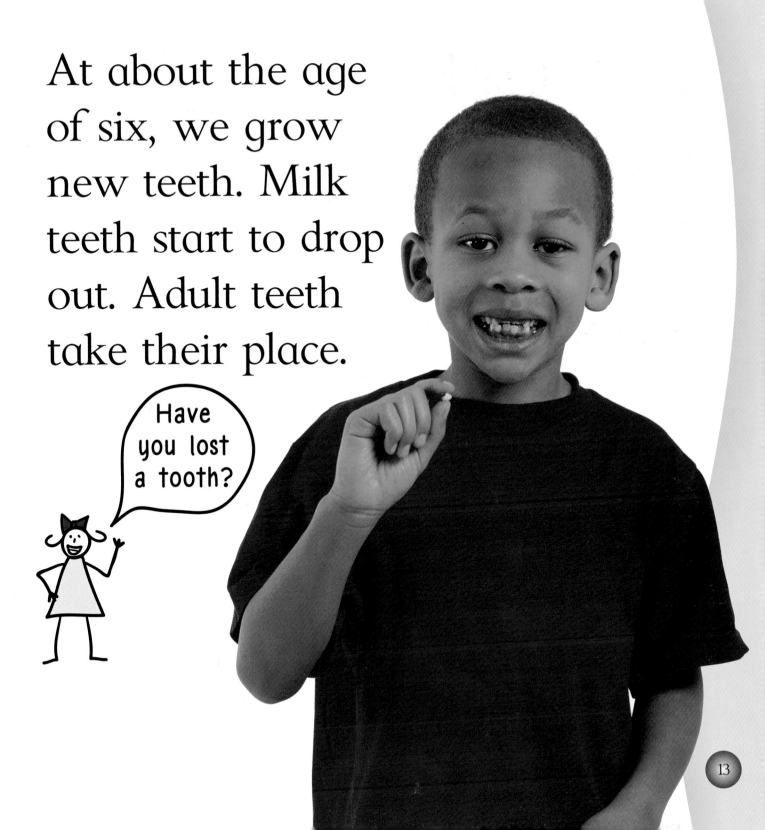

Adult teeth

By the time we are 18 years old, we have a full set of 32 teeth.

How many teeth do you have?

Canines (cutting teeth)

Incisors (cutting teeth)

Molars (flat teeth for chewing)

Premolars (teeth between canines and molars)

Adult teeth are big and strong, and have to last a lifetime.

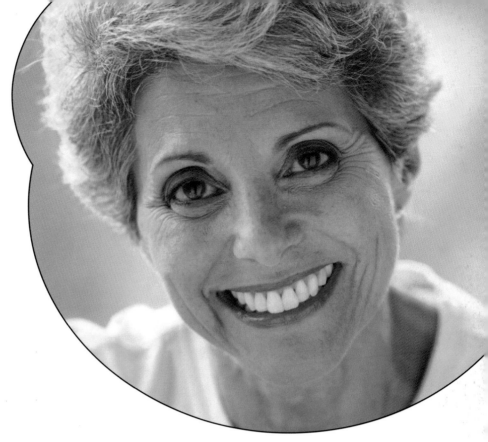

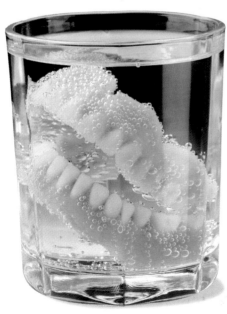

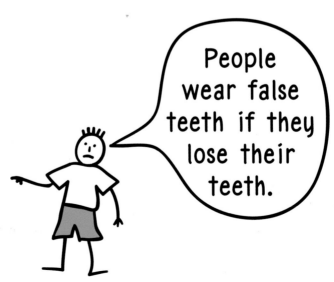

People wear false teeth if they lose their teeth.

Food can harm teeth

Many foods contain sugar. It mixes with germs to attack our teeth.

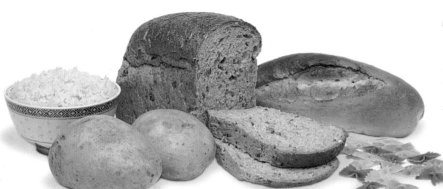

These foods release sugar as we chew them.

These contain sugar.

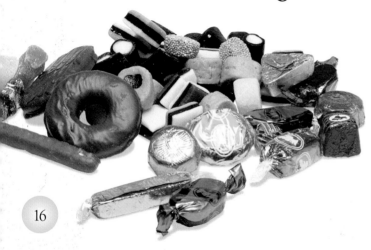

These contain natural sugar.

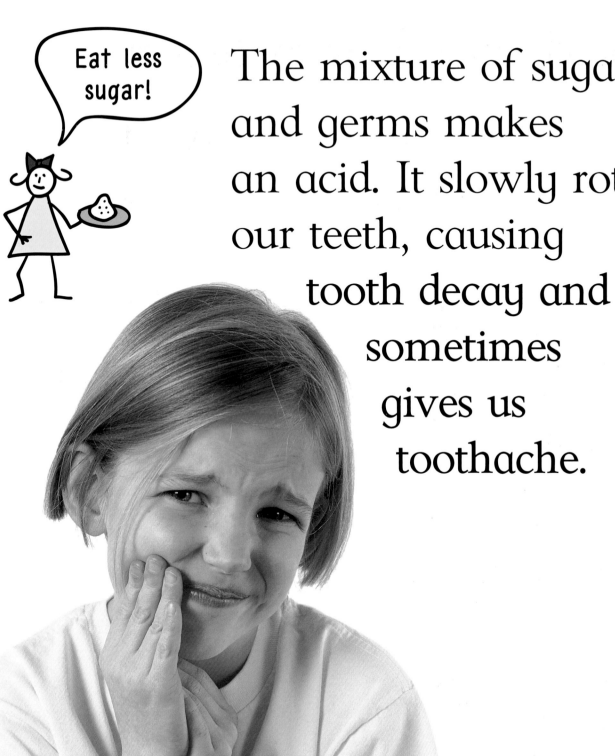

Eat less sugar!

The mixture of sugar and germs makes an acid. It slowly rots our teeth, causing tooth decay and sometimes gives us toothache.

Brushing your teeth

Brushing your teeth helps get rid of the germs and sugar.

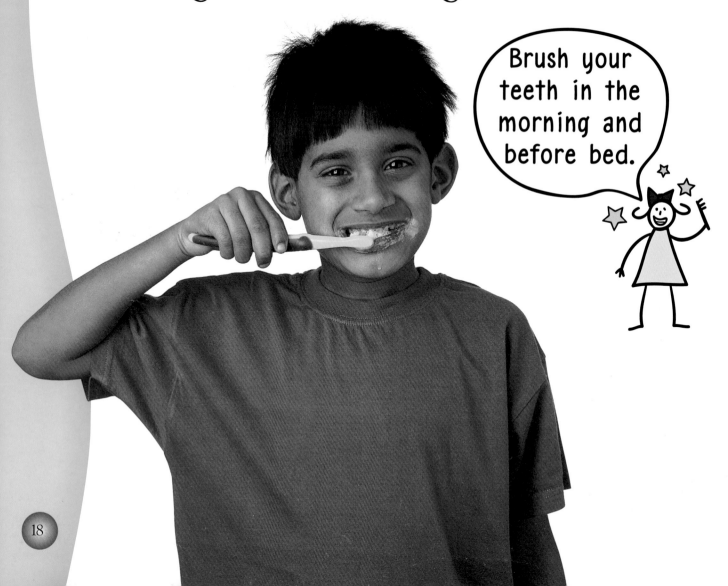

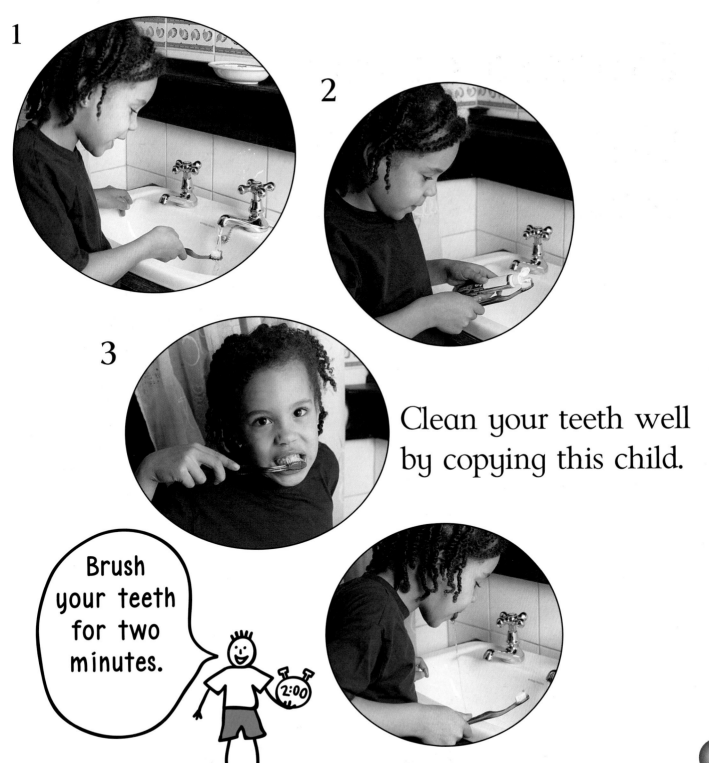

1

2

3

Clean your teeth well by copying this child.

Brush your teeth for two minutes.

Cutting down on sugar

You can protect your teeth by eating fewer sugary foods.

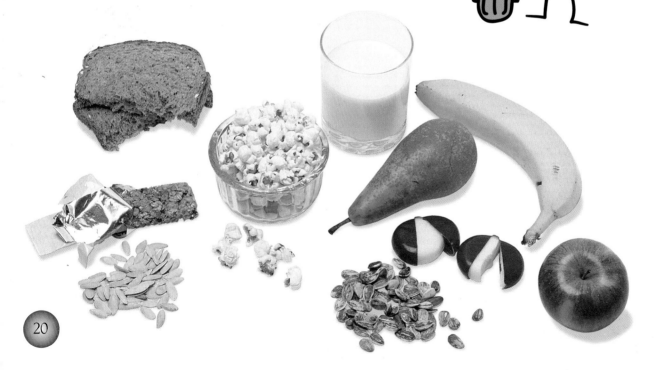

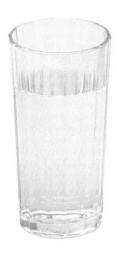

Water is the best drink for your teeth. We all like to eat sweet foods sometimes. Try to eat them only at meals.

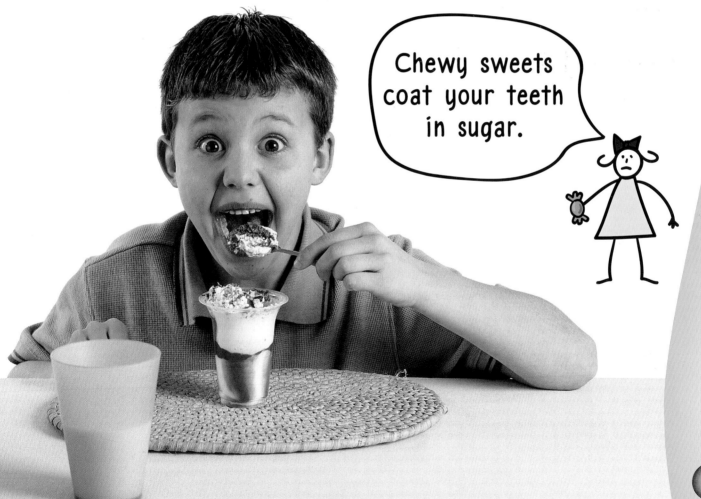

Chewy sweets coat your teeth in sugar.

Going to the dentist

Dentists check that your teeth are growing well and are being cleaned properly.

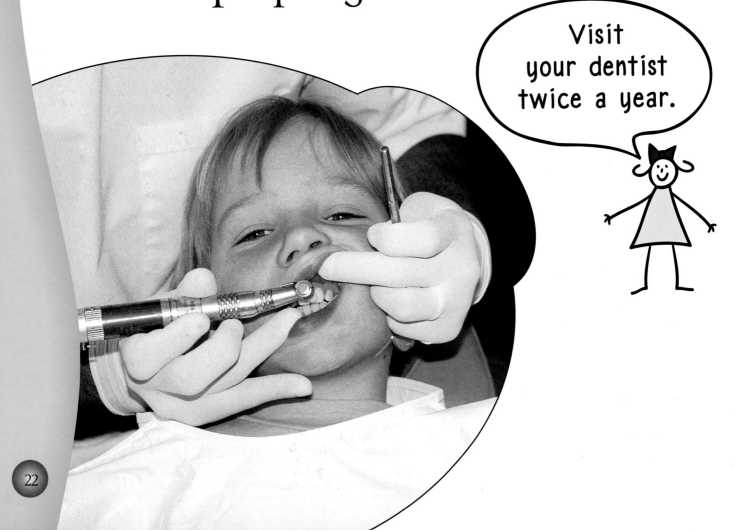

Visit your dentist twice a year.

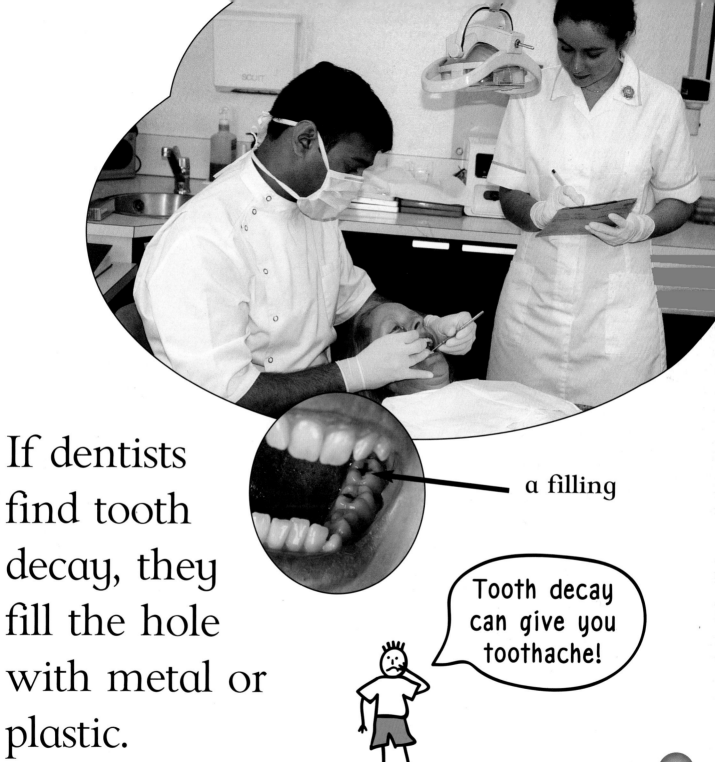

If dentists find tooth decay, they fill the hole with metal or plastic.

a filling

Tooth decay can give you toothache!

A helping hand

Sometimes teeth need to be straightened by braces.

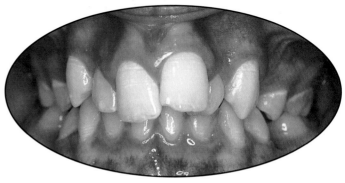

1 Crooked teeth

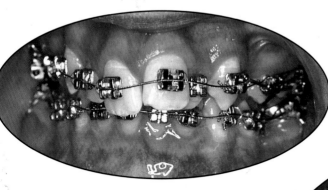

2 Braces are fitted

3 Straightened teeth

Wearing braces helps push the teeth gently into place. Dentists can also repair chipped teeth.

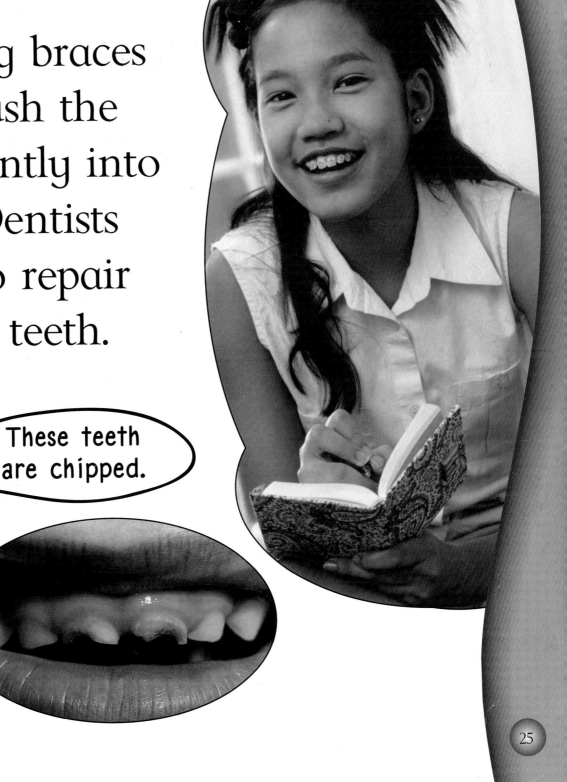

These teeth are chipped.

Healthy teeth

Everyone wants healthy teeth. Eating some foods, like milk and cheese, helps make teeth stronger.

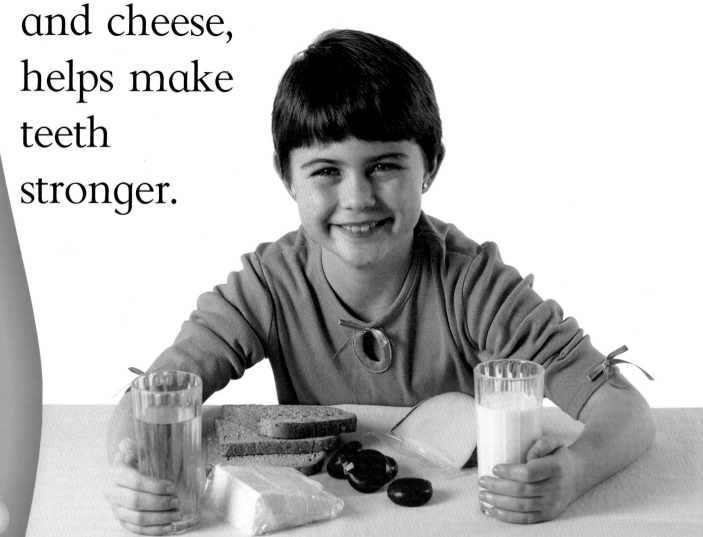

Here are three ways to
look after your teeth:

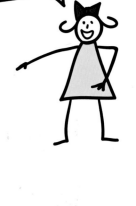

Say 'No' to sweets!

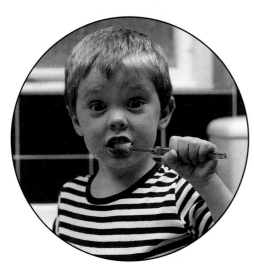

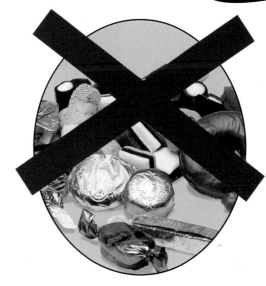

1 Brush
your teeth
twice a
day.

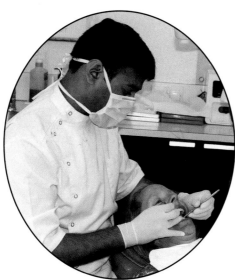

2 Have fewer
sugary foods
and drinks.

3 Visit your
dentist twice
a year.

Glossary

acid A strong substance that attacks teeth.

adult teeth The second set of teeth that replaces the milk teeth. They are never replaced.

braces A wire frame used to straighten teeth.

enamel The hard, white coating on the outside of a tooth.

filling The metal or plastic that dentists use to fill a hole caused by tooth decay.

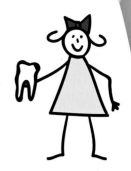

germs Tiny living things that ar around us. Some cause tooth decay.

gum The part of the mouth that helps hold the teeth in the jaw.

milk teeth The small first teeth that come through when we are babies and are replaced by our adult teeth.

root The part of the tooth that grows inside the gum.

swallow To move food or drink from the mouth and into the throat.

tooth decay When teeth rot and develop holes.

Index

About this book

Learning the principles of how to keep healthy and clean is one of life's most important skills. **Let's Get Healthy** is a series aimed at young children who are just beginning to develop these skills. **Your Teeth** looks at our teeth and how to care for them.

Here are a number of activities that children could try:

Pages 6-7 Use (clean!) fingers to feel their own teeth. How many do they have? What do they feel like?

Pages 8-9 Discuss how gums are just as important as the teeth themselves — the gums hold the teeth in place, and if they are not looked after properly, the teeth will fall out.

Pages 10-11 Identify each kind of tooth in their own mouths. Make a list of different foods and decide which teeth are used for eating each one (it may be more than one kind).

Pages 12-13 Do a survey of how many milk teeth each child has. Compare this with their ages.

Pages 14-15 Discuss why children have milk teeth (their jaws are too small for adult teeth).

Pages 16-17 Use disclosing tablets to find where plaque has built up.

Pages 18-19 Make teeth 'dirty' by eating some chocolate. What's the best way to clean them? Try rinsing with water, using the tongue and brushing them.

Pages 20-21 Collect the packaging for different soft drinks. Which ones have the highest sugar content?

Pages 22-23 Make a poster to encourage children to go to the dentist.

Pages 24-25 Discuss reasons why it's usually necessary to straighten crooked teeth and repair broken ones (to make it easier to eat, speak or to keep them healthy).

Pages 26-27 Think up some recipes that contain foods that will help build strong teeth.

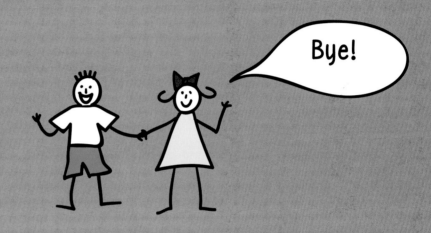